Renal

Diet 101

How to Strengthen Kidney Health
and Shed Pounds Fast and Easy With
Incredible Kidney-Friendly Recipes
for Everyday Cooking

Aileen Horton

TABLE OF CONTENTS

INTRODUCTION

For your diabetic family and friends, you'll find recipes for tasty, nutritious, low-carbohydrate, high-protein meals. This cookbook will help patients explore new foods that are appropriate for their kidney nutrition while keeping track of their food intake. Each menu includes easy-to-read nutritional facts, as well as kidney-friendly recipes and meals created by chefs and nutritionists to be suitable for kidney nutrition.

Kidney dieticians have accepted low salt kidney-friendly recipes for patients with kidney disease, kidney dysfunction, and chronic kidney failure. Look for kidney meal ideas to feed patients with chronic kidney failure and other kidney issues. Create a low-salt kidney meal by making salads, making essential amino acids, and making a sandwich with this recipe.

This is a lunch suggestion for kidney nutrients, plus it's high in potassium, so you may imagine it'll help you choose foods like apricots, potatoes, and raisins. This is an example of a diet meal schedule that can assist you with making eating decisions. Recipes for kidney patients with progressive kidney disorder and kidney dysfunction that are low in salt. potassium deficiency Low-salt, low-sodium, high-protein

Kidney flour alternatives include low-sodium, sodium-free vanilla cans.

I've sifted through tens of thousands of recipes to find all of the diabetic kidney diet recipes you'll ever need. We sift through the millions of food ideas you've taken with you from all over the world, as well as some of the most common recipes on the Internet. They sift through millions of recipes from around the world to offer you a variety of diabetic and kidney-friendly recipes that you must try.

We provide recipes, magazines, and counselors to help kidney patients and their families take care of themselves. Magical ginger cookies for the holidays can be found in the Kidney Kitchen e-News, which has been certified by a kidney dietitian, as well as several other online cookbooks.

Nothing beats a vegetarian diet for keeping the kidneys in good shape, and it's been shown that following a kidney diet doesn't have to be boring or bland. This handy cookbook contains 100 basic kidney diets - nutritious recipes to get you started. To help a balanced kidney, get all of your kidney diet recipes, including breakfast, lunch, dinner, snacks, and drinks.

And if it puts you at risk, a low-salt, low-fat diet helps you deal with the kind of diet that can carry you to your bones. Remember to eat high-quality, high-protein foods after you've figured out which foods are healthy for kidney nutrition and which are poor. MagicKitchen.com has all of your kidney recipes, and they're full of taste and versatility thanks to new herbs, tomatoes, whole grains, almonds, beans, fruits, and vegetables.

Patients with kidney disease should follow the kidney dietary recommendations to the letter, but following a kidney diet to the letter can be difficult. This list of kidney nutrient meals will make life simpler for you and your colleagues, as well as kidney disease patients. It can be difficult to keep track of a kidney disorder. Following a kidney disease diet can be difficult, so this list of kidney-fed meals can make it a lot easier.

BREAKFAST

1. Fine Morning Porridge

Preparation Time: 15 minutes

Cooking Time: 10 minutes

Servings: 2

Ingredients:

- 2 tablespoons coconut flour
- 2 tablespoons vanilla protein powder
- 3 tablespoons Golden Flaxseed meal
- 1 ½ cups almond almond milk, unsweetened
- Powdered erythritol

Directions:

1. Take a bowl and mix in flaxseed meal, protein powder, coconut flour and mix well
2. Add mix to the saucepan (placed over medium heat)
3. Add almond almond milk and stir, let the mixture thicken
4. Add your desired amount of sweetener and serve

Nutrition: Calories: 259 Fat: 13g Carbohydrates: 5g Protein: 16g

2. Hungarian's Porridge

Preparation Time: 10 minutes

Cooking Time: 10 minutes

Servings: 2

Ingredients:

- 1 tablespoon chia seeds
- 1 tablespoon ground flaxseed
- 1/3 cup coconut cream
- ½ cup of water
- 1 teaspoon vanilla extract
- 1 tablespoon almond butter

Directions:

1. Add chia seeds, coconut cream, flaxseed, water and vanilla to a small pot
2. Mix and let it sit for 6 minutes
3. Put butter and place pot over low heat
4. Keep stirring as butter melts
5. Once the porridge is hot/not boiling, pour into a bowl
6. Add a few berries or a dash of cream for extra flavor

Nutrition: Calories: 410 Fat: 38g Carbohydrates: 10g Protein: 6g

3. Zucchini and Onion Platter

Preparation Time: 15 minutes

Cooking Time: 45 minutes

Servings: 4

Ingredients:

- 3 large zucchinis, julienned
- ½ cup basil
- 2 red onions, thinly sliced
- ¼ teaspoon salt
- 1 teaspoon cayenne pepper
- 2 tablespoons lemon juice

Directions:

1. Create zucchini Zoodles by using a vegetable peeler and shaving the zucchini with peeler lengthwise until you get to the core and seeds
2. Turn zucchini and repeat until you have long strips
3. Discard seeds
4. Lay strips on cutting board and slice lengthwise to your desired thickness
5. Mix Zoodles in a bowl alongside onion, basil, and toss
6. Sprinkle salt and cayenne pepper on top
7. Drizzle lemon juice

Nutrition: Calories: 156 Fat: 8g Carbohydrates: 6g Protein: 7g

4. Chorizo and Egg Tortilla

Preparation Time: 10 minutes

Cooking Time: 13 minutes

Servings: 1 tortilla

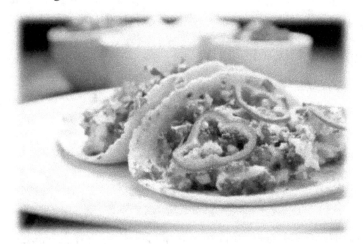

Ingredients:

- 1 flour tortilla, about 6-inches
- 1/3 cup chorizo meat, chopped
- 1 egg

Directions:

1. Take a medium-sized skillet pan, place it over medium heat and when hot, add chorizo.

2. When the meat has cooked, drain the excess fat, whisk an egg, pour it into the pan, stir until combined, and cook for 3 minutes, or until eggs have cooked.

3. Spoon egg onto the tortilla and then serve.

Nutrition: Calories – 223 Fat – 11 g Protein – 16 g Carbohydrates – 15 g Fiber – 1.5 g

5. Cottage Pancakes

Preparation Time: 10 minutes

Cooking Time: 50 minutes

Servings: 6 pancakes

Ingredients:

- 3 cups fresh raspberries, sliced
- ½ cup all-purpose white flour
- 6 tablespoons unsalted butter, melted
- 4 eggs, beaten

Directions:

1. Crack eggs in a medium-sized bowl, add flour, and butter in it, and whisk until combined.

2. Take a medium-high frying pan, grease it with oil and when hot, pour in prepared batter, ¼ cup of batter per pancake, spread the batter into a 4-inch pancake, and cook for 3 minutes per side until browned.

3. When done, transfer pancakes onto a plate, cook more pancakes in the same manner, and, when done, serve each pancake with ½ sliced raspberries.

Nutrition: Calories – 253 Fat – 17 g Protein – 11 g Carbohydrates – 21 g Fiber – 2 g

6. Egg in a Hole

Preparation Time: 5 minutes

Cooking Time: 5 minutes

Servings: 1 slice

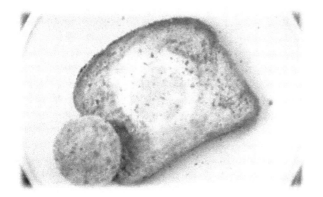

Ingredients:

- 1 slice of white bread
- ¼ teaspoon lemon pepper seasoning, salt-free
- 1 egg

Directions:

1. Prepare the bread by making a hole in the middle: use a cookie cutter for cutting out the center.

2. Brush the slice with oil on both sides, then take a medium-sized skillet pan, place it over medium heat and when hot, add bread slice in it, crack the egg in the center of the slice sprinkle with lemon pepper seasoning.

3. Cook the egg for 2 minutes, then carefully flip it along with the slice and continue cooking for an additional 2 minutes.

Nutrition: Calories – 159 Fat – 7 g Protein – 9 g Carbohydrates – 15 g Fiber – 0.8 g

7. German Pancakes

Preparation Time: 10 minutes

Cooking Time: 15 minutes

Servings: 10 pancakes

Ingredients:

- 2/3 cup all-purpose flour
- ¼ teaspoon vanilla extract, unsweetened
- 2 tablespoons white sugar
- 1 cup almond milk, low-fat
- 4 eggs
- 1/3 cup fruit jam for serving, sugar-free

Directions:

1. Prepare the batter by taking a medium-sized bowl, add flour in it along with sugar, stir until mixed, whisk in eggs until blended, and then whisk in vanilla and almond milk until smooth.

2. Take a skillet pan, about 8 inches, spray it with oil and when hot, add 3 tablespoons of the prepared batter, tilt the pan to spread the batter evenly

3. Flip the pancake, continue cooking for 45 seconds until the other side is browned, and when done, transfer pancake to a plate.

4. Cook nine more pancakes in the same manner and, when done on one side of the pancake, fold it, and then serve with 1 tablespoon of fruit jam.

Nutrition: Calories – 74 Fat – 2 g Protein – 4 g Carbohydrates – 10 g Fiber – 0.2 g

LUNCH

8. Ground Beef and Bell Peppers

Preparation Time: 10 minutes

Cooking Time: 10 minutes

Serving: 3

Ingredients:

- 1 onion, chopped
- 2 tablespoons coconut oil
- 1-pound ground beef
- 1 red bell pepper, diced
- 2 cups green lettuce, chopped
- Salt and pepper to taste

Directions:

1. Place over medium heat on a skillet
2. Add onion and cook until slightly browned
3. Add green lettuce and ground beef
4. Stir fry until done
5. Take the mixture and fill up the bell peppers
6. Serve and enjoy!

Nutrition: Calories: 350 Fat: 23g Carbohydrates: 4g Protein: 28g

9. Spiced Up Pork Chops

Preparation Time: 4 hours 10 minutes

Cooking Time: 15 minutes

Serving: 4

Ingredients:

- ¼ cup lime juice
- 4 pork rib chops
- 1 tablespoon coconut oil, melted
- 2 garlic cloves, peeled and minced
- 1 tablespoon chili powder
- 1 teaspoon ground cinnamon
- 2 teaspoons cumin
- Salt and pepper to taste
- ½ teaspoon hot pepper sauce
- Mango, sliced

Directions:

1. Take a bowl and mix in lime juice, oil, garlic, cumin, cinnamon, chili powder, salt, pepper, hot pepper sauce
2. Whisk well
3. Add pork chops and toss
4. Keep it on the side and refrigerate for 4 hours
5. Pre-heat your grill to medium and transfer pork chops to a pre-heated grill
6. Grill for 7 minutes both sides
7. Divide between serving platters and serve with mango slices

8. Enjoy!

Nutrition: Calories: 200 Fat: 8g Carbohydrates: 3g Protein: 26g

10. Juicy Salmon Dish

Preparation Time: 5 minutes

Cooking Time: 6 minutes

Serving: 3

Ingredients:

- ¾ cup of water
- Few sprigs of parsley, basil, tarragon, basil
- 1 pound of salmon, skin on
- 3 teaspoons of ghee
- ¼ teaspoon of salt
- ½ teaspoon of pepper
- ½ of lemon, thinly sliced
- 1 whole carrot, julienned

Directions:

1. Set your pot to Sauté mode and add water and herbs
2. Place a steamer rack inside your pot and place salmon
3. Drizzle ghee on top of the salmon and season with salt and pepper
4. Cover with lemon slices
5. Cook on HIGH pressure with locked lid for 3 minutes
6. Release the pressure naturally over 10 minutes
7. Transfer the salmon to a serving platter
8. Set your pot to Sauté mode and add vegetables
9. Cook for 1-2 minutes
10. Serve with vegetables and salmon
11. Enjoy!

Nutrition Values: Calories: 464 Fat: 34g Carbohydrates: 3g Protein: 34g

DINNER

11. Sautéed Butternut Squash

Preparation Time: 25 minutes

Cooking Time: 10 minutes

Servings: 8

Ingredients:

- 1 tbsp. of oil, olive
- 4 cups of peeled, de-seeded, cubed squash, butternut
- 1/2 chopped onion, sweet
- 1 tsp. of chopped thyme, fresh
- A pinch pepper, ground

Directions:

1. Heat oil in large-sized skillet on med-high heat.
2. Add squash. Sauté till tender, 15-17 minutes.
3. Add thyme and onion. Sauté for five minutes more.
4. Season using ground pepper. Serve while hot.

Nutrition: For each serving (1 serving) 50 calories 1.5 g fat 0 mg cholesterol 8 g carbs 2 g sugar 2 g fiber 2 g protein 3 mg sodium 36 mg calcium 20 mg phosphorus 243 mg potassium

12. Herb Roasted Chicken

Preparation Time: 25 minutes

Cooking Time: 20 minutes

Servings: 4

Ingredients:

- 1 lb. of chicken breasts, skinless, boneless
- 1 onion, medium
- 1 or 2 cloves of garlic, fresh
- 2 tbsp. of herb & garlic seasoning
- 1 tsp. of pepper, ground
- 1/4 cup of oil, olive

Directions:

1. Chop the garlic and onion. Place in bowl. Add oil, seasoning and pepper.
2. Add chicken to marinade and cover. Then, place in refrigerator for four hours or overnight.
3. Preheat oven to 375F.
4. Cover cookie sheet with aluminum foil. Place marinated chicken on foil.
5. Pour remainder of marinade over chicken. Bake in 375F oven for 18-20 minutes.
6. Broil for five extra minutes to brown, if desired. Serve.

Nutrition: For each serving (4 ounces) 268 calories 16 g fat 82 mg cholesterol 52 mg sodium 2 g carbs 25 g protein 250 mg phosphorus 489 mg potassium 0.5 g fiber 16 mg calcium

13. Seared Scallops

Preparation Time: 25 minutes

Cooking Time: 20 minutes

Servings: 4

Ingredients:

- 1 tbsp. of oil, olive
- 12 oz. of rinsed, patted dry sea scallops
- Pepper, ground, as desired
- 2 tbsp. of lemon juice, freshly squeezed if available
- 1 tsp. each of fresh chopped parsley, thyme and chives

Directions:

1. Heat oil in large-sized skillet on med-high.
2. Season scallops lightly using pepper. Add to skillet.
3. Sea scallops and turn once till just cooked fully through and lightly browned, three to four minutes.
4. Add and stir in lemon juice, chives, parsley and thyme.
5. Turn scallops, coating in herb sauce. Serve while hot.

Nutrition: For each serving (3 scallops) 119 calories 4 g fat 26 mg cholesterol 2 g carbs 0 g sugar 4 g fiber 12 g protein 288 mg sodium 7 mg calcium 245 mg phosphorus 199 mg potassium

14. Greek Salad

Preparation Time: 10 minutes

Cooking time: 0 minutes

Servings: 2 servings

Ingredients:

- 2 cups lettuce leaves
- 2 cucumbers
- 1 tablespoon lemon juice
- 1 teaspoon olive oil
- ¼ teaspoon dried oregano
- ½ teaspoon salt
- ¼ teaspoon chili flakes
- 4 oz. Feta cheese

Directions:

1. Chop Feta cheese into the small cubes.
2. Chop the lettuce leaves roughly put them in the salad bowl.
3. Then chop cucumbers into the cubes. Add them in the lettuce bowl.
4. For the dressing: whisk together chili flakes, salt, dried oregano, olive oil, and lemon juice.
5. Pour the dressing over the lettuce mixture and mix up well.

6. Sprinkle the salad with Feta cubes and shake gently.

Nutrition: Calories 312, fat 21.2, fiber 5.3, carbs 23.5, protein 11.9

MAIN DISHES

15. Cream Cheese Salmon Toast

Preparation Time: 15 minutes

Cooking Time: 5 minutes

Servings: 2

Ingredients:

- Whole grain or rye toast, two slices
- 1 tbsp. Red onion, chopped fine
- 2 tbsp. Cream cheese, low-fat
- ½ tsp. Basil flakes
- ½ cup Arugula or spinach, chopped
- 2 oz. Smoked salmon

Directions:

1. Toast the wheat bread. Mix cream cheese and basil and spread this mixture on the toast. Add salmon, arugula, and onion.

Nutrition: Calories 291 15.2 grams fat (8.5 saturated) 17.8 grams carbohydrates 3 grams of sugar

16. Carrot Cake Overnight Oats

Preparation Time: 5 minutes + overnight

Cooking Time: 0 minutes

Servings: 1

Ingredients:

- 1 cup Coconut or almond milk
- 1 tbsp. Chia seeds
- 1 tsp. Cinnamon, ground
- ½ cup Raisins
- 2 tbsp. Cream cheese, low fat, at room temperature
- 1 Large Carrot, peel, and shred
- 2 tbsp. Honey
- 1 tsp. Vanilla

Directions:

1. Mix together all of the listed ingredients and store them in a safe refrigerator container overnight. Eat cold in the morning. If you choose to warm this, just microwave for one minute and stir well before eating.

Nutrition: Calories 340 32 grams sugar 8 grams protein 4 grams fat 9 grams fiber 70 grams carbs

17. Mediterranean Frittata

Preparation Time: 5 minutes

Cooking Time: 20 minutes

Servings: 6

Ingredients:

- 6 Eggs
- ¼ cup Feta cheese, crumbled
- ¼ tsp. Black pepper
- Oil, spray or olive
- 1 tsp. Oregano
- ¼ cup Almond milk, almond or coconut
- 1 tsp. Sea salt
- ¼ cup Black capers, chopped
- ¼ cup Green capers, chopped
- ¼ cup Bell pepper, diced

Directions:

1. Heat oven to 400. Oil one eight by eight-inch baking dish. Beat the almond milk into the eggs, and then add other ingredients. Pour all of this mixture into the baking dish and bake for twenty minutes.

Nutrition: Calories 107 2 grams sugars 7 fat grams 3 carb grams 7 grams protein

SNACKS

18. Sweet and spicy tortilla chips

Preparation time: 10 minutes

Cooking time: 8 minutes

Servings: 6

Ingredients

- 1/4 cup butter
- 1 teaspoon brown sugar
- 1/2 teaspoon ground chili powder
- 1/2 teaspoon garlic powder
- 1/2 teaspoon ground cumin
- 1/4 teaspoon ground cayenne pepper
- 6 flour tortillas, 6" size

Directions

1. Preheat oven to 425 degrees f.
2. Grease a baking sheet with cooking spray.
3. Add all spices, brown sugar, and melted butter to a small bowl.
4. Mix well and set this mixture aside.
5. Slice the tortillas into 8 wedges and brush them with the sugar mixture.

6. Spread them on the baking sheet and bake them for 8 minutes.

7. Serve fresh.

Nutrition: calories 115. Protein 2 g. Carbohydrates 11 g. Fat 7 g. Cholesterol 15 mg. Sodium 156 mg. Potassium 42 mg. Phosphorus 44 mg. Calcium 31 mg. Fiber 0.6 g.

19. Addictive pretzels

Preparation time: 10 minutes

Cooking time: 1 hour

Servings: 6

Ingredients

- 32-ounce bag unsalted pretzels
- 1 cup canola oil
- 2 tablespoon seasoning mix
- 3 teaspoon garlic powder
- 3 teaspoon dried dill weed

Directions

1. Preheat oven to 175 degrees f.
2. Place the pretzels on a cooking sheet and break them into pieces.
3. Mix garlic powder and dill in a bowl and reserve half of the mixture.
4. Mix the remaining half with seasoning mix and ¾ cup of canola oil.
5. Pour this oil over the pretzels and brush them liberally
6. Bake the pieces for 1 hour then flip them to bake for another 15 minutes.
7. Allow them to cool then sprinkle the remaining dill mixture and drizzle more oil on top.
8. Serve fresh and warm.

Nutrition: calories 184. Protein 2 g. Carbohydrates 22 g. Fat 8 g. Cholesterol 0 mg. Sodium 60 mg. Potassium 43 mg. Phosphorus 28 mg. Calcium 2 mg. Fiber 1.0 g.

20. Shrimp spread with crackers

Preparation time: 10 minutes

Cooking time: 0 minutes

Servings: 6

Ingredients

- 1/4 cup light cream cheese
- 2 1/2-ounce cooked, shelled shrimp, minced
- 1 tablespoon no-salt-added ketchup
- 1/4 teaspoon hot sauce
- 1 teaspoon worcestershire sauce
- 1/2 teaspoon herb seasoning blend
- 24 matzo cracker miniatures
- 1 tablespoon parsley

Directions

1. Start by tossing the minced shrimp with cream cheese in a bowl.
2. Stir in worcestershire sauce, hot sauce, herb seasoning, and ketchup.
3. Mix well and garnish with minced parsley.
4. Serve the spread with the crackers.

Nutrition: calories 57. Protein 3 g. Carbohydrates 7 g. Fat 1 g. Cholesterol 21 mg. Sodium 69 mg. Potassium 54 mg. Phosphorus 30 mg. Calcium 15 mg. Fiber 0.2 g.

21. Buffalo chicken dip

Preparation time: 10 minutes

Cooking time: 3 hours

Servings: 4

Ingredients

- 4-ounce cream cheese
- 1/2 cup bottled roasted red peppers
- 1 cup reduced-fat sour cream
- 4 teaspoon hot pepper sauce
- 2 cups cooked, shredded chicken

Directions

1. Blend half cup of drained red peppers in a food processor until smooth.
2. Now, thoroughly mix cream cheese, and sour cream with the pureed peppers in a bowl.
3. Stir in shredded chicken and hot sauce then transfer the mixture to a slow cooker.
4. Cook for 3 hours on low heat.
5. Serve warm with celery, carrots, cauliflower, and cucumber.

Nutrition: calories 73. Protein 5 g. Carbohydrates 2 g. Fat 5 g. Cholesterol 25 mg. Sodium 66 mg. Potassium 81 mg. Phosphorus 47 mg. Calcium 31 mg. Fiber 0 g.

SOUP AND STEW

22. Lemony Lentil Salad with Salmon

Preparation time: 10 minutes

Cooking time: 0 minutes

Servings: 3

Ingredients:

- ¼ tsp salt
- ½ cup chopped red onion
- 1 cup diced seedless cucumber
- 1 medium red bell pepper, diced
- 1/3 cup extra virgin olive oil
- 1/3 cup fresh dill, chopped
- 1/3 cup lemon juice
- 2 15oz cans of lentils
- 2 7oz cans of salmon, drained and flaked
- 2 tsp Dijon mustard
- Pepper to taste

Directions:

1. In a bowl, mix, lemon juice, mustard, dill, salt and pepper. Gradually add the oil, bell pepper, onion, cucumber, salmon flakes and lentils. Toss to coat evenly.

Nutrition: calories 450, fat 22 g, fiber 10 g, carbs 62 g, protein 55 g

23. Spaghetti Squash & Yellow Bell-Pepper Soup

Preparation Time: 10 minutes

Cooking Time: 45 minutes

Servings: 4

Ingredients:

- 2 diced yellow bell peppers
- 2 chopped large garlic cloves
- 1 peeled and cubed spaghetti squash
- 1 quartered and sliced onion
- 1 tbsp. dried thyme
- 1 tbsp. coconut oil
- 1 tsp. curry powder
- 4 cups water

Directions:

2. Heat the oil in a large pan over medium-high heat before sweating the onions and garlic for 3-4 minutes.
3. Sprinkle over the curry powder.
4. Add the stock and bring to a boil over a high heat before adding the squash, pepper and thyme.
5. Turn down the heat, cover and allow to simmer for 25-30 minutes.
6. Continue to simmer until squash is soft if needed.
7. Allow to cool before blitzing in a blender/food processor until smooth.
8. Serve!

Nutrition: Calories 103, Protein 2 g, Carbs 17 g,Fat 4 g, Sodium (Na) 32 mg, Potassium (K)365 mg,Phosphorus 50 mg

24. Red Pepper & Brie Soup

Preparation Time: 10 minutes

Cooking Time: 35 minutes

Servings: 4

Ingredients:

- 1 tsp. paprika
- 1 tsp. cumin
- 1 chopped red onion
- 2 chopped garlic cloves
- ¼ cup crumbled brie
- 2 tbsps. extra virgin olive oil
- 4 chopped red bell peppers
- 4 cups water

Directions:

1. Heat the oil in a pot over medium heat.
2. Sweat the onions and peppers for 5 minutes.
3. Add the garlic cloves, cumin and paprika and sauté for 3-4 minutes.
4. Add the water and allow to boil before turning the heat down to simmer for 30 minutes.
5. Remove from the heat and allow to cool slightly.
6. Put the mixture in a food processor and blend until smooth.
7. Pour into serving bowls and add the crumbled brie to the top with a little black pepper.
8. Enjoy!

Nutrition: Calories 152, Protein 3 g, Carbs 8 g, Fat 11 g, Sodium (Na) 66 mg, Potassium (K) 270 mg, Phosphorus 207 mg

25. Turkey & Lemon-Grass Soup

Preparation Time: 5 minutes

Cooking Time: 40 minutes

Servings: 4

Ingredients:

- 1 fresh lime
- ¼ cup fresh basil leaves
- 1 tbsp. cilantro
- 1 cup chestnuts
- 1 tbsp. coconut oil
- 1 thumb-size minced ginger piece
- 2 chopped scallions
- 1 finely chopped green chili
- 4oz. skinless and sliced turkey breasts
- 1 minced garlic clove, minced
- ½ finely sliced stick lemon-grass
- 1 chopped white onion, chopped
- 4 cups water

Directions:

1. Crush the lemon-grass, cilantro, chili, 1 tbsp oil and basil leaves in a blender or pestle and mortar to form a paste.
2. Heat a large pan/wok with 1 tbsp olive oil on high heat.
3. Sauté the onions, garlic and ginger until soft.
4. Add the turkey and brown each side for 4-5 minutes.
5. Add the broth and stir.

6. Now add the paste and stir.
7. Next add the chestnuts, turn down the heat slightly, and simmer for 25-30 minutes or until turkey is thoroughly cooked through.
8. Serve hot with the green onion sprinkled over the top.

Nutrition: Calories 123, Protein 10 g, Carbs 12 g, Fat 3 g, Sodium (Na) 501 mg, Potassium (K) 151 mg, Phosphorus 110 mg

26. Paprika pork soup

Preparation time:5 minutes

Cooking time:35 minutes

Servings:2

Ingredients

- 4-ounce sliced pork loin
- 1 teaspoon black pepper
- 2 minced garlic cloves
- 3 cups water
- 1 tablespoon extra-virgin olive oil
- 1 chopped onion
- 1 tablespoon paprika

Directions

1. Add in the oil, chopped onion and minced garlic.
2. Sauté for 5 minutes on low heat.
3. Add the pork slices to the onions and cook for 7-8 minutes or until browned.
4. Add the water to the pan and bring to a boil on high heat.
5. Reduce heat and simmer for a further 20 minutes or until pork is thoroughly cooked through.
6. Season with pepper to serve.

Nutrition: calories 165, protein 13 g, carbs 10 g, fat 9 g, sodium (na) 269 mg, potassium (k) 486 mg, phosphorus 158 mg

VEGETABLE

27. Steamed Collard Greens

Preparation Time: 10 minutes

Cooking Time: 5 minutes

Servings: 2

Ingredients:

- 2 cups Collard Greens
- 1 tablespoon lime juice
- 1 teaspoon olive oil
- 1 teaspoon sesame seeds
- ½ teaspoon chili flakes
- 1 cup water, for the steamer

Directions:

1. Chop collard greens roughly.
2. Pour water in the steamer and insert rack.
3. Place the steamer bowl, add collard greens, and close the lid.
4. Steam the greens for 5 minutes.
5. After this, transfer the steamed collard greens in the salad bowl.
6. Sprinkle it with the lime juice, olive oil, sesame seeds, and chili flakes.
7. Mix up greens with the help of 2 forks and leave to rest for 10 minutes before serving.

Nutrition: Calories 43, Fat 3.4, Fiber 1.7, Carbs 3.4, Protein 1.3

28. Baked Eggplants Slices

Preparation Time: 15 minutes

Cooking Time: 15 minutes

Servings: 3

Ingredients:

- 1 large eggplant, trimmed
- 1 tablespoon butter, softened
- 1 teaspoon minced garlic
- 1 teaspoon salt

Directions:

1. Slice the eggplant season it with salt. Mix up well and leave for 10 minutes to make the vegetable "give" bitter juice.
2. After this, dry the eggplant with the paper towel.
3. In the shallow bowl, mix up together minced garlic and softened butter.
4. Brush every eggplant slice with the garlic mixture.
5. Line the baking tray with baking paper. Preheat the oven to 355F.
6. Place the sliced eggplants in the tray to make 1 layer and transfer it in the oven.
7. Bake the eggplants for 15 minutes. The cooked eggplants will be tender but not soft!

Nutrition: Calories 81, Fat 4.2, Fiber 6.5,Carbs 11.1, Protein 1.9

29. Vegetable Masala

Preparation Time: 10 minutes

Cooking Time: 18 minutes

Servings: 4

Ingredients:

- 2 cups green beans, chopped
- 1 cup white mushroom, chopped
- ¾ cup Red bell peppers, crushed
- 1 teaspoon minced garlic
- 1 teaspoon minced ginger
- 1 teaspoon chili flakes
- 1 tablespoon garam masala
- 1 tablespoon olive oil
- 1 teaspoon salt

Directions:

1. Line the tray with parchment and preheat the oven to 360F.
2. Place the green beans and mushrooms in the tray.
3. Sprinkle the vegetables with crushed Red bell peppers, minced garlic and ginger, chili flakes, garam masala, olive oil, and salt.
4. Mix up well and transfer in the oven.
5. Cook vegetable masala for 18 minutes.

Nutrition: Calories 60, Fat 30.7, Fiber 2.5, Carbs 6.4, Protein 2

SIDE DISHES

30. Cauliflower Patties

Preparation Time: 5 minutes

Cooking Time: 8 minutes

Servings: 4

Ingredients:

- Eggs – 2
- Egg whites – 2
- Onion – ½, diced
- Cauliflower – 2 cups, frozen
- All-purpose white flour – 2 Tbsps.
- Black pepper – 1 tsp.
- Coconut oil – 1 Tbsp.
- Curry powder – 1 tsp.
- Fresh cilantro – 1 Tbsp.

Directions:

1. Soak vegetables in warm water before cooking.
2. Steam cauliflower over a pan of boiling water for 10 minutes.
3. Blend eggs and onion in a food processor before adding cooked cauliflower, spices, cilantro, flour, and pepper and blast in the processor for 30 seconds.
4. Heat a skillet on a high heat and add oil.
5. Enjoy with a salad.

Nutrition: Calories: 227 Fat: 12g Carb: 15g Phosphorus: 193mg Potassium: 513mg Sodium: 158mg Protein: 13g

SALAD

31. Barb's Asian Slaw

Preparation Time: 5 minutes

Cooking Time: 5 minutes

Servings: 2

Ingredients:

- 1 cabbage head, shredded
- 4 chopped green onions
- ½ cup slivered or sliced almonds
- Dressing:
- ½ cup olive oil
- ¼ cup tamari or soy sauce
- 1 tablespoon honey or maple syrup
- 1 tablespoon baking stevia

Directions:

1. Heat up dressing ingredients in a saucepan on the stove until thoroughly mixed.
2. Mix all ingredients when you are ready to serve.

Nutrition: Calories: 205 Protein: 27g Carbohydrate: 12g Fat: 10 g Calcium 29mg, Phosphorous 76mg, Potassium 27mg Sodium: 111 mg

FISH & SEAFOOD

32. Fish Tacos

Preparation Time: 10 minutes

Cooking Time: 35 minutes

Servings: 6

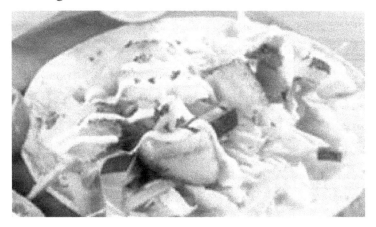

Ingredients:

- 1½ cup of cabbage
- ½ cup of red onion
- ½ bunch of cilantro
- 1 garlic clove
- 2 limes
- 1 pound of cod fillets
- ½ teaspoon of ground cumin
- ½ teaspoon of chili powder
- ¼ teaspoon of black pepper
- 1 tablespoon of olive oil

- ½ cup of mayonnaise
- ¼ cup of sour cream
- 2 tablespoons of almond milk
- 12 (6-inch) corn tortillas

Directions:

1. Shred the cabbage, chop the onion and cilantro, and mince the garlic. Set aside
2. Use a dish to place in the fish fillets, then squeeze half a lime juice over the fish. Sprinkle the fish fillets with the minced garlic, cumin, black pepper, chili powder, and olive oil. Turn the fish filets to coat with the marinade, then refrigerate for about 15 to 30 minutes
3. Prepare salsa Blanca by mixing the mayonnaise, almond milk, sour cream, and the other half of the lime juice. Stir to combine, then place in the refrigerator to chill
4. Broil in oven, and cover the broiler pan with aluminum foil. Broil the coated fish fillets for about 10 minutes or until the flesh becomes opaque and white and flakes easily. Remove from the oven, slightly cool, and then flake the fish into bigger pieces
5. Heat the corn tortillas in a pan, one at a time until it becomes soft and warm, then wrap in a dish towel to keep them warm
6. To assemble the tacos, place a piece of the fish on the tortilla, topping with the salsa blanca, cabbage, cilantro, red onion, and the lime wedges.
7. Serve with hot sauce if you desire

Nutrition: Calories 363 Protein 18g Carbohydrates 30g Fat 19g Cholesterol 40mg Sodium 194mg Potassium 507mg Phosphorus 327mg Fiber 4.3g

33. Jambalaya

Preparation Time: 10 minutes

Cooking Time: 1 hour and 15 minutes

Servings: 12

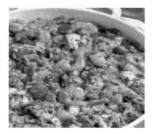

Ingredients:

- 2 cups of onion
- 1 cup of bell pepper
- 2 garlic cloves
- 2 cups of uncooked converted white rice
- ½ teaspoon of black pepper
- 8 ounces of canned low-sodium tomato sauce
- 2 cups of low-sodium beef broth
- 2 pounds of raw shrimp
- ½ cup of unsalted margarine

Directions:

1. Preheat oven to 350º F
2. Chop the onion, bell pepper, garlic, then peel the shrimp
3. Combine and mix all the ingredients in a large bowl except the margarine

4. Pour into a 9 x 13-inch baking dish and evenly spread out
5. Slice the margarine, placing over the top of the ingredients
6. Cover with foil or lid, and bake for about 1 hr 15 minutes
7. Serve hot.

Nutrition: Calories 294 Protein 20g Carbohydrates 31g Fat 10g Cholesterol 137mg Sodium 186mg Potassium 300mg Phosphorus 197mg Fiber 0.8g

34. Asparagus Shrimp Linguini

Preparation Time: 10 minutes

Cooking Time: 35 minutes

Servings: 1 ½ cup

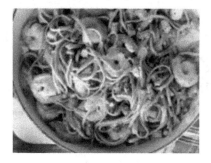

Ingredients:

- 8 ounces of uncooked linguini
- 1 tablespoon of olive oil
- 1¾ cups of asparagus
- ½ cup of unsalted butter
- 2 garlic cloves
- 3 ounces of cream cheese
- 2 tablespoons of fresh parsley
- ¾ teaspoon of dried basil
- 2/3 cup of dry white wine
- ½ pound of peeled and cooked shrimp

Directions:

1. Preheat oven to 350° F
2. Cook the linguini in boiling water until it becomes tender, then drain

3. Place the asparagus on a baking sheet, then spread two tablespoons of oil over the asparagus. Bake for about 7 to 8 minutes or until it is tender
4. Remove baked asparagus from the oven and place it on a plate. Cut the asparagus into pieces of medium-sized once cooled
5. Mince the garlic and chop the parsley
6. Melt ½ cup of butter in a large skillet with the minced garlic
7. Stir in the cream cheese, mixing as it melts
8. Stir in the parsley and basil, then simmer for about 5 minutes. Mix either in boiling water or dry white wine, stirring until the sauce becomes smooth
9. Add the cooked shrimp and asparagus, then stir and heat until it is evenly warm
10. Toss the cooked pasta with the sauce and serve

Nutrition: Calories 544 Protein 21g Carbohydrates 43g Fat 32g Cholesterol 188mg Sodium 170mg Potassium 402mg Phosphorus 225mg Fiber 2.4g

35. Tuna Noodle Casserole

Preparation Time: 10 minutes

Cooking Time: 35 minutes

Servings: 2

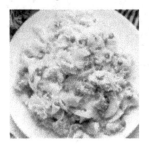

Ingredients:

- 2 ounces of wide uncooked egg noodles
- 5 ounces of canned tuna in water
- ½ cup of sour cream
- ¼ cup of cottage cheese
- ½ cup of fresh sliced mushrooms
- ½ cup of frozen green peas
- 1 tablespoon of unsalted butter
- ¼ cup of unseasoned bread crumbs

Directions:

1. Preheat oven to 350° F
2. Boil egg noodles based on the package instructions and drain. Also, drain and flake the tuna
3. Combine and mix the sour cream, cottage cheese, mushrooms, tuna, and peas in a medium bowl

4. Stir the drained noodle into the tuna mixture, and place in a small casserole dish that has been sprayed with a non-stick cooking spray
5. Melt butter, stir into the bread crumbs, then sprinkle over the mixture of noodles in step 4
6. Bake for about 20 to 25 minutes or until the bread crumbs start to brown
7. Divide into two and serve

Nutrition: Calories 415 Protein 22g Carbohydrates 39g Fat 19g Cholesterol 88mg Sodium 266mg Potassium 400mg Phosphorus 306mg Fiber 3.2g

36. Oven-Fried Southern Style Catfish

Preparation Time: 10 minutes

Cooking Time: 35 minutes

Servings: 4

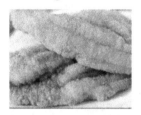

Ingredients:

- 1 egg white
- ½ cup of all-purpose flour
- ¼ cup of cornmeal
- ¼ cup of panko bread crumbs
- 1 teaspoon of salt-free Cajun seasoning
- 1 pound of catfish fillets

Directions:

1. Heat oven to 450° F
2. Use cooking spray to spray a non-stick baking sheet
3. Using a bowl, beat the egg white until very soft peaks are formed. Don't over-beat
4. Use a sheet of wax paper and place the flour over it
5. Using a different sheet of wax paper to combine and mix the cornmeal, panko and the Cajun seasoning
6. Cut the catfish fillet into four pieces, then dip the fish in the flour, shaking off the excess

7. Dip coated fish in the egg white, rolling into the cornmeal mixture
8. Place the fish on the baking pan. Repeat with the remaining fish fillets
9. Use cooking spray to spray over the fish fillets. Bake for about 10 to 12 minutes or until the sides of the fillets become browned and crisp

Nutrition: Calories 250 Protein 22g Carbohydrates 19g Fat 10g Cholesterol 53mg Sodium 124mg Potassium 401mg Phosphorus 262mg Fiber 1.2g

POULTRY RECIPES

37. Ground Chicken with Basil

Preparation Time: 15 minutes

Cooking Time: 16 minutes

Servings: 8

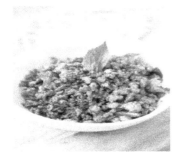

Ingredients:

- 2 pounds lean ground chicken
- 3 tablespoons coconut oil, divided
- 1 zucchini, chopped
- 1 red bell pepper, seeded and chopped
- ½ of green bell pepper, seeded and chopped
- 4 garlic cloves, minced
- 1 (1-inch) piece fresh ginger, minced
- 1 (1-inch) piece fresh turmeric, minced
- 1 fresh red chili, sliced thinly
- 1 tablespoon organic honey
- 1 tablespoon coconut aminos
- 1½ tablespoons fish sauce
- ½ cup fresh basil, chopped

- Salt
- ground black pepper
- 1 tablespoon fresh lime juice

Directions:

1. Heat a large skillet on medium-high heat. Add ground beef and cook for approximately 5 minutes or till browned completely.
2. Transfer the beef to a bowl. In a similar pan, melt 1 tablespoon of coconut oil on medium-high heat. Add zucchini and bell peppers and stir fry for around 3-4 minutes.
3. Transfer the vegetables inside the bowl with chicken. In precisely the same pan, melt remaining coconut oil on medium heat. Add garlic, ginger, turmeric, and red chili and sauté for approximately 1-2 minutes.
4. Add chicken mixture, honey, and coconut aminos and increase the heat to high. Cook within 4-5 minutes or till sauce is nearly reduced. Stir in remaining ingredients and take off from the heat.

Nutrition: Calories: 407 Fat: 7g Carbohydrates: 20g Fiber: 13g Protein: 36g Phosphorus 149 mg Potassium 706.3 mg Sodium 21.3 mg

38. Chicken &Veggie Casserole

Preparation Time: 15 minutes

Cooking Time: 30 minutes

Servings: 4

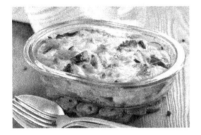

Ingredients:

- 1/3 cup Dijon mustard
- 1/3 cup organic honey
- 1 teaspoon dried basil
- ¼ teaspoon ground turmeric
- 1 teaspoon dried basil, crushed
- Salt
- ground black pepper
- 1¾ pound chicken breasts
- 1 cup fresh white mushrooms, sliced
- ½ head broccoli, cut into small florets

Directions:

1. Warm oven to 350 degrees F. Lightly greases a baking dish. In a bowl, mix all ingredients except chicken, mushrooms, and broccoli.

2. Put the chicken in your prepared baking dish, then top with mushroom slices. Place broccoli florets around chicken evenly.
3. Pour 1 / 2 of honey mixture over chicken and broccoli evenly. Bake for approximately 20 minutes. Now, coat the chicken with the remaining sauce and bake for about 10 minutes.

Nutrition: Calories: 427 Fat: 9g Carbohydrates: 16g Fiber: 7g Protein: 35g Phosphorus 353 mg Potassium 529.3 mg Sodium 1 mg

39. Chicken & Cauliflower Rice Casserole

Preparation Time: 15 minutes

Cooking Time: 1 hour & 15 minutes

Servings: 8-10

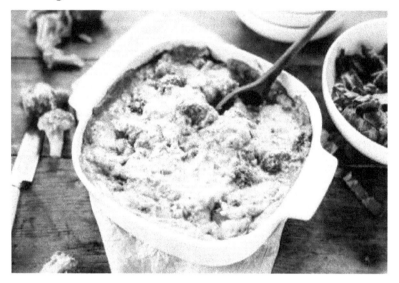

Ingredients:

- 2 tablespoons coconut oil, divided
- 3-pound bone-in chicken thighs and drumsticks
- Salt
- ground black pepper
- 3 carrots, peeled and sliced
- 1 onion, chopped finely
- 2 garlic cloves, chopped finely
- 2 tablespoons fresh cinnamon, chopped finely
- 2 teaspoons ground cumin
- 1 teaspoon ground coriander
- 12 teaspoon ground cinnamon

- ½ teaspoon ground turmeric
- 1 teaspoon paprika
- ¼ tsp red pepper cayenne
- 1 (28-ounce) can diced Red bell peppers with liquid
- 1 red bell pepper, thin strips
- ½ cup fresh parsley leaves, minced
- Salt, to taste
- 1 head cauliflower, grated to some rice-like consistency
- 1 lemon, sliced thinly

Directions:

1. Warm oven to 375 degrees F. In a large pan, melt 1 tablespoon of coconut oil at high heat. Add chicken pieces and cook for about 3-5 minutes per side or till golden brown.
2. Transfer the chicken to a plate. In a similar pan, sauté the carrot, onion, garlic, and ginger for about 4-5 minutes on medium heat.
3. Stir in spices and remaining coconut oil. Add chicken, Red bell peppers, bell pepper, parsley plus salt, and simmer for approximately 3-5 minutes.
4. In the bottom of a 13x9-inch rectangular baking dish, spread the cauliflower rice evenly. Place chicken mixture over cauliflower rice evenly and top with lemon slices.
5. With foil paper, cover the baking dish and bake for approximately 35 minutes. Uncover the baking dish and bake for about 25 minutes.

Nutrition: Calories: 412 Fat: 12g Carbohydrates: 23g Protein: 34g Phosphorus 201 mg Potassium 289.4 mg Sodium 507.4 mg

40. Chicken Meatloaf with Veggies

Preparation Time: 20 minutes

Cooking Time: 1-1¼ hours

Servings: 4

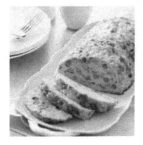

Ingredients:

- For Meatloaf:
- ½ cup cooked chickpeas
- 2 egg whites
- 2½ teaspoons poultry seasoning
- Salt
- ground black pepper
- 10-ounce lean ground chicken
- 1 cup red bell pepper, seeded and minced
- 1 cup celery stalk, minced
- 1/3 cup steel-cut oats
- 1 cup tomato puree, divided
- 2 tablespoons dried onion flakes, crushed
- 1 tablespoon prepared mustard
- For Veggies:
- 2-pounds summer squash, sliced
- 16-ounce frozen Brussels sprouts

- 2 tablespoons extra-virgin extra virgin olive oil
- Salt
- ground black pepper

Directions:

1. Warm oven to 350 degrees F. Grease a 9x5-inch loaf pan. In a mixer, add chickpeas, egg whites, poultry seasoning, salt, and black pepper and pulse till smooth.
2. Transfer a combination in a large bowl. Add chicken, veggies oats, ½ cup of tomato puree, and onion flakes and mix till well combined.
3. Transfer the amalgamation into the prepared loaf pan evenly. With both hands, press down the amalgamation slightly.
4. In another bowl, mix mustard and remaining tomato puree. Place the mustard mixture over the loaf pan evenly.
5. Bake approximately 1-1¼ hours or till the desired doneness. Meanwhile, in a big pan of water, arrange a steamer basket. Cover and steam for about 10-12 minutes. Drain well and aside.
6. Now, prepare the Brussels sprouts according to the package's directions. In a big bowl, add veggies, oil, salt, and black pepper and toss to coat well. Serve the meatloaf with veggies.

Nutrition: Calories: 420 Fat: 9g Carbohydrates: 21g Protein: 36g Phosphorus 237.1 mg Potassium 583.6 mg Sodium 136 mg

MEAT RECIPES

41. Baked Pork & Mushroom Meatballs

Preparation Time: 15 minutes

Cooking Time: fifteen minutes

Servings: 6

Ingredients:

- 1-pound lean ground pork
- 1 organic egg white, beaten
- 4 fresh shiitake mushrooms, stemmed and minced
- 1 tablespoon fresh parsley, minced
- 1 tablespoon fresh basil leaves, minced
- 1 tablespoon fresh mint leaves, minced
- 2 teaspoons fresh lemon zest, grated finely
- 11/2 teaspoons fresh ginger, grated finely
- Salt and freshly ground black pepper, to taste

Directions:

1. Preheat the oven to 425 degrees F. Arrange the rack inside center of oven.
2. Line a baking sheet with a parchment paper.
3. In a sizable bowl, add all ingredients and mix till well combined.
4. Make small equal-sized balls from mixture.

5. Arrange the balls onto prepared baking sheet in a single layer.

6. Bake for approximately 12-15 minutes or till done completely.

Nutrition: Calories: 411, Fat: 19g, Carbohydrates: 27g, Fiber: 11g, Protein: 35g

42. Beef Ragu

Preparation Time: 10 minutes

Cooking Time: 10 minutes

Servings: 2

Ingredients:

- 1/4 cup packaged pesto
- 1 teaspoon salt
- 2 large zucchinis, cut into noodle strips
- 1 tablespoon olive oil
- 1/4-pound ground beef
- 4 tablespoons fresh parsley, chopped

Directions:

1. Heat the oil in a skillet under medium flame and cook the ground beef until thoroughly cooked, around 5 minutes. Discard excess fat.

2. Add the packaged pesto sauce and season with salt. Add t

3. Then chopped parsley and cook for three more minutes. Set aside.

4. In the same saucepan, place the zucchini noodles and cook for five minutes. Turn off the heat then add the cooked meat. Mix well.

5. Serve and enjoy.

Nutrition: Calories 353, Total Fat 30g, Saturated Fat 6g, Total Carbs 2g, Net Carbs 1.3g, Protein 19g, Sugar: 0.3g, Fiber 0.7g, Sodium 1481mg, Potassium 341mg

Broths, Condiment And Seasoning

43. Poultry Seasoning Mix

Preparation Time: 15 minutes

Cooking Time: 0 minutes

Servings: 2 tbsp.

Ingredients:

- 2 teaspoons dried thyme leaves
- 2 teaspoons dried basil leaves
- 1½ teaspoons dried marjoram leaves
- ¼ teaspoon onion powder
- ¼ teaspoon garlic powder
- 1/8 teaspoon freshly ground black pepper

Directions:

1. Combine the thyme, basil, marjoram, onion powder, garlic powder, and pepper in a small bowl and mix. Store at room temperature. You can grind all of these ingredients together to make a more like commercial poultry seasoning.

Nutrition: Calories: 21 Fat: >1g Sodium: 23mg Potassium: 132mg Phosphorus: 17mg Carbohydrates: 5g Protein: 1g

44. Homemade Mustard

Preparation Time: 15 minutes

Cooking Time: 0 minutes

Servings: ½ cup

Ingredients:

- ¼ cup dry mustard
- 3 tablespoons mustard seeds
- 3 tablespoons apple cider vinegar
- 3 tablespoons water
- 2 tablespoons freshly squeezed lemon juice
- ½ teaspoon turmeric

Directions:

1. Combine the dry mustard, mustard seeds, vinegar, water, lemon juice, and turmeric in a jar with a tight-fitting lid and stir to combine.
2. Refrigerate the mustard for 3 days, stirring once a day and adding a bit more water every day if necessary.
3. After three days, the mustard is ready to use. You can process the mixture in a food processor or blender if you'd like smoother mustard. Refrigerate up to 2 weeks.

Nutrition: Calories: 9 Fat: 0g Sodium: 0mg Potassium: 16mg Phosphorus: 13mg Carbohydrates: 1g Protein: 0g

45. Cranberry Ketchup

Preparation Time: 15 minutes

Cooking Time: 20 minutes

Servings: 1 cup

Ingredients:

- 2 cups fresh cranberries
- 1 1/3 cups water
- 3 tablespoons brown sugar
- Juice of 1 lemon
- 2 teaspoons yellow mustard
- ¼ teaspoon onion powder
- Pinch salt
- Pinch ground cloves

Directions:

1. Stir together the cranberries, water, brown sugar, lemon juice, mustard, onion powder, salt, and cloves in a medium saucepan on medium heat, then boil.
2. Reduce the heat to low and simmer until the cranberries have popped, about 15 minutes. Mash using an immersion blender the ingredients right in the saucepan.
3. After mashing, simmer the ketchup for another 5 minutes until thickened. Let the ketchup cool for 1 hour in the saucepan, then put it into an airtight container and store.

Nutrition: Calories: 13 Fat: 0g Sodium: 19mg Potassium: 17mg Phosphorus: 3mg Carbohydrates: 3g Protein: 0g

DRINKS AND SMOOTHIES

46. Blueberry Smoothie

Preparation Time: 5 minutes

Cooking Time: 2 minutes

Servings: 4

Ingredients:

- 1 c. frozen blueberries
- 6 tbsp. protein powder
- 8 packets Splenda
- 14 oz. apple juice, unsweetened
- 8 cubes of ice

Directions:

1. Take a blender and place all the ingredients (in order) in it. process for 1 minute until smooth.
2. Distribute the smoothie between four glasses and then serve.

Nutrition: Calories: 162 Fat: 0.5g Carbs: 30g Protein: 8g Sodium: 123.4mg Potassium: 223mg Phosphorus: 109mg

47. Blackberry Sage Cocktail

Preparation Time: 5 minutes

Cooking Time: 10 minutes

Servings: 6

Ingredients:

- Sage Simple Syrup
- 1 cup water
- 1 cup0granulated sugar
- 8 fresh sage leaves, plus more for garnish
- 1-pint fresh blackberries, muddled and strained (juices reserved)
- Juice of 1/2 a lemon
- 8 oz St. Germain Liqueur
- 16 oz vodka
- seltzer water

Directions:

1. Place water and sugar in a small saucepan.
2. Simmer until sugar dissolves for 7 to 10 minutes.
3. Remove from heat. Add sage leaves, and cover, allowing the mixture for about 2 hours.
4. Combine fresh blackberry juice, lemon juice, sage simple syrup, cocktail pitcher.
5. Mix and refrigerate covered until well chilled.

6. Serve in cocktail glasses filled with ice and garnish with fresh sage leaves and top with a splash of seltzer water.

Nutrition: Calories: 68 Fat: 1g Carbs: 15g Protein: 3g Sodium: 3mg Potassium: 133mg Phosphorus: 38mg

DESSERT

48. Healthy Cinnamon Lemon Tea

Preparation Time: 5 minutes

Cooking Time: 5 minutes

Servings: 1

Ingredients:

- 1/2 tbsp fresh lemon juice
- 1 cup of water
- 1 tsp ground cinnamon

Directions:

1. Add water in a saucepan and bring to boil over medium heat.

2. Add cinnamon and stir to cinnamon dissolve.

3. Add lemon juice and stir well.

4. Serve hot.

Nutrition: Calories 9 Fat 0.2 g Carbohydrates 2 g Sugar 0.3 g Protein 0.2 g Cholesterol 0 mg Phosphorus: 70mg Potassium: 87mg Sodium: 65mg

49. Keto Mint Ginger Tea

Preparation Time: 5 minutes

Cooking Time: 5 minutes

Servings: 1

Ingredients:

- 1 1/2 tbsp fresh mint leaves

- 1 cup of water

- 1/2 tbsp fresh ginger, grated

- 1 tsp ground turmeric

Directions:

1. Add mint, ginger, and turmeric in boiling water.

2. Stir to turmeric dissolved.

3. Strain and serve.

Nutrition: Calories 19 Fat 0.3 g Carbohydrates 4 g Sugar 0.3 g Protein 0.5 g Cholesterol 0 mg Phosphorus: 110mg Potassium: 117mg Sodium: 75mg

50. Energy Booster Sunflower Balls

Preparation Time: 10 minutes

Cooking Time: 10 minutes

Servings: 25

Ingredients:

- 1 cup sunflower seeds
- 2 oz unsweetened chocolate, melted
- 1 tbsp water
- 8 drops liquid stevia

Directions:

1. Add sunflower seeds in a blender and blend until finely ground.
2. Add water, stevia, and melted chocolate and blend until stiff dough like the mixture is form.
3. Make small balls from mixture and place on a baking tray.
4. Place in refrigerator for 30 minutes.
5. Serve and enjoy.

Nutrition: Calories 22 Fat 2.1 g Carbohydrates 1.1 g Sugar 0.1 g Protein 0.7 g Cholesterol 0 mg Phosphorus: 130mg Potassium: 127mg Sodium: 95mg

51. Mixed Berries Crisp

Preapration Time:10 Minutes

Cooking Time:: 12 Minutes

Serves 4

Ingredients:

- 1/2cup fresh blueberries
- 1/2cup chopped fresh strawberries
- 1/3cup frozen raspberries, thawed
- 1 tablespoon honey
- 1 tablespoon freshly squeezed lemon juice
- ⅔ cup whole-wheat pastry flour
- 3 tablespoons packed brown sugar
- 2 tablespoons unsalted butter, melted

Directions:

1. Place the strawberries, blueberries, and raspberries in a baking pan and drizzle the honey and lemon juice over the top.
2. Combine the pastry flour and brown sugar in a small mixing bowl.
3. Add the butter and whisk until the mixture is crumbly. Scatter the flour mixture on top of the fruit.
4. Place the pan on the bake position.
5. Set Time to 12 minutes.
6. When cooking is complete, the fruit should be bubbly and the topping should be golden brown.

Nutrition: Calories: 170 Carbs: 8 g Fat: 6 g Protein: 16 g

52. Duck Fat Roasted Red Potatoes

Preapration Time:5 minutes

Cooking Time: 25 minutes

Servings: 4

Ingredients:

- 4 red potatoes, cut into wedges
- 1 tbsp. garlic powder
- 2 tbsp. thyme, chopped
- 3 tbsp. duck fat, melted

Directions:

1. Preheat air fryer to 380 F. In a bowl, mix duck fat, garlic powder, salt, and pepper. Add the potatoes and shake to coat.
2. Place in the basket and bake for 12 minutes, remove the basket, shake and continue cooking for another 8-10 minutes until golden brown. Serve warm topped with thyme.

Nutrition: Calories: 110 Carbs: 8 g Fat: 5 g Protein: 7 g

53. Chicken Wings with Alfredo Sauce

Preapration Time:5 minutes

Cooking Time: 20 minutes

Servings: 4

Ingredients:

- 1 1/2 lb. chicken wings, pat-dried
- Salt to taste
- 1/2 cup Alfredo sauce

Directions:

1. Season the wings with salt. Arrange them in the greased air fryer basket, without touching and AirFry for 12 minutes until no longer pink in the center. Work in batches if needed. Flip them, increase the heat to 390 F and cook for 5 more minutes. Plate the wings and drizzle with Alfredo sauce to serve.

Nutrition: Calories: 150 Carbs: 7 g Fat: 5 g Protein: 14 g

54. Crispy Squash

Preapration Time:5 minutes

Cooking Time: 20 minutes

Servings: 4

Ingredients:

- 2 cups butternut squash, cubed
- 2 tbsp. olive oil
- Salt and black pepper to taste
- ¼ tsp. dried thyme
- 1 tbsp. fresh parsley, finely chopped

Directions:

1. In a bowl, add squash, olive oil, salt, pepper, thyme, and toss to coat.
2. Place the squash in the air fryer and Air Fry for 14 minutes at 360 F, shaking once or twice. Serve sprinkled with fresh parsley.

Nutrition: Calories: 100 Carbs: 5 g Fat: 2 g Protein: 3 g

55. Classic French Fries

Preapration Time:5 minutes

Cooking Time: 30 minutes

Servings: 4

Ingredients

- (2 servings)
- 2 russet potatoes, cut into strips
- 2 tbsp. olive oil
- Kosher salt and black pepper to taste
- 1/2 cup aioli

Directions::

1. Preheat the fryer to 400 F. Spray the air fryer basket with cooking spray.
2. In a bowl, brush the strips with olive oil and season with salt and black pepper. Put it in the air fryer and cook for 20-22 minutes, turning once halfway through, until crispy. Serve with garlic aioli.

Nutrition: Calories: 120 Carbs: 7 g Fat: 4 g Protein: 6 g

56. BBQ Chicken

Preapration Time:5 minutes

Cooking Time: 30 minutes

Servings: 4

Ingredients:

- 1 whole small chicken, cut into pieces
- 1 tsp. salt
- 1 tsp. smoked paprika
- 1 tsp. garlic powder
- 1 cup BBQ sauce

Directions:

1. Mix salt, paprika, and garlic powder and coat the chicken pieces. Place in the air fryer basket and Bake for 18 minutes at 400 F. Remove to a plate and brush with barbecue sauce.
2. Wipe the fryer clean from the chicken fat. Return the chicken to the fryer, skin-side up, and Bake for 5 more minutes at 340 F.

Nutrition: Calories: 230 Carbs: 12 g Fat: 9 g Protein: 23 g

57. Turkey Meatballs with Spaghetti Squash

Preapration Time:15 minutes

Cooking Time: 35 minutes

Servings: 4

Ingredients:

- 1 lb. lean ground turkey
- 1 lb. spaghetti squash, halved and seeds removed
- 2 egg whites
- 1/3 cup green onions, diced fine
- ¼ cup onion, diced fine
- 2 ½ tbsp. flat leaf parsley, diced fine
- 1 tbsp. fresh basil, diced fine
- What you'll need from store cupboard:
- 14 oz. can no-salt-added tomatoes, crushed
- 1/3 cup soft whole wheat bread crumbs
- ¼ cup low sodium chicken broth
- 1 tsp garlic powder
- 1 tsp thyme
- 1 tsp oregano
- ½ tsp red pepper flakes
- ½ tsp whole fennel seeds

Directions:

1. In a small bowl, combine bread crumbs, onion, garlic, parsley, pepper flakes, thyme, and fennel.

2. In a large bowl, combine turkey and egg whites. Add bread crumb mixture and mix well. Cover and chill 10 minutes. Heat the oven to broil.
3. Place the squash, cut side down, in a glass baking dish. Add 3-4 tablespoons of water and microwave on high 10-12 minutes, or until fork tender.
4. Make 20 meatballs from the turkey mixture and place on a baking sheet. Broil 4-5 minutes, turn and cook 4 more minutes.
5. In a large skillet, combine tomatoes and broth and bring to a simmer over low heat. Add meatballs, oregano, basil, and green onions. Cook, stirring occasionally, 10 minutes or until heated through.
6. Use a fork to scrape the squash into "strands" and arrange on a serving platter. Top with meatballs and sauce and serve.

Nutrition: Calories 253 Total Carbs 15g Net Carbs 13g Protein 27g Fat 9g Sugar 4g Fiber 2g

58. Turkey & Mushroom Casserole

Preapration Time:15 minutes

Cooking Time: 50 minutes

Servings: 8

Ingredients:

- 1 lb. cremini mushrooms, washed and sliced
- 1 onion, diced
- 6 cup cauliflower, grated
- 4 cup turkey, cooked and cut in bite size pieces
- 2 cup reduced fat Mozzarella, grated, divided
- 1 cup fat free sour cream
- ½ cup lite mayonnaise
- ¼ cup reduced fat parmesan cheese
- 2 tbsp. olive oil, divided
- 2 tbsp. Dijon mustard
- 1 ½ tsp thyme
- 1 ½ tsp poultry seasoning

Directions:

1. Heat oven to 375 degrees. Spray a 9x13-inch baking dish with cooking spray.
2. In a medium bowl, stir together sour cream, mayonnaise, mustard, ½ teaspoon each thyme and poultry seasoning, 1 cup of the mozzarella, and parmesan cheese.
3. Heat 2 teaspoons oil in a large skillet over med-high heat. Add mushrooms and sauté until they start to

brown and all liquid is evaporated. Transfer them to the Directions:ared baking dish.

4. Add 2 more teaspoons oil to the skillet along with the onion and sauté until soft and they start to brown. Add the onions to the mushrooms.

5. Add another 2 teaspoons oil to the skillet with the cauliflower. Cook, stirring frequently, until it starts to get soft, about 3-4 minutes. Add the remaining thyme and poultry seasoning and cook 1 more minute.

6. Season with salt and pepper and add to baking dish. Place the turkey over the vegetables and stir everything together.

7. Spread the sauce mixture over the top and stir to combine. Sprinkle the remaining mozzarella over the top and bake 40 minutes, or until bubbly and cheese is golden brown. Let cool 5 minutes, then cut and serve.

Nutrition: Calories 351 Total Carbs 13g Net Carbs 10g Protein 37g Fat 16g Sugar 5g Fiber 3g

59. Prosciutto-Wrapped Asparagus

Preapration Time:10 m

Cooking Time 12 m

6 Servings

Ingredients:

- 12 spears asparagus, trimmed
- 2 teaspoons olive oil
- Salt and freshly ground black pepper, to taste
- 12 prosciutto slices

Directions::

1. Drizzle the asparagus spears with oil and ten, sprinkle with salt and black pepper.
2. Wrap one prosciutto slice around each asparagus spear from top to bottom.
3. Turn the "Temperature Knob" of PowerXL Air Fryer Grill to line the temperature to 300 degrees F.
4. Turn the "Function Knob" to settle on "Air Fry."
5. Turn the "Timer Knob" to line the Time for 10 minutes.
6. After preheating, arrange the asparagus spears into the greased air fry basket.
7. Insert the air fry basket at position 2 of the Air Fryer Grill.
8. Flip the asparagus spears once halfway through.
9. When the cooking Time is over, transfer the asparagus spears onto a platter.
10. Serve hot.

Nutrition: Calories: 144 Kcal, Fat: 8.7g, Carb: 1.9g, Protein: 16g

60. Coconut Shrimp

Preapration Time:15 m

Cooking Time 8 m

3 Servings

Ingredients:

- ¼ cup almond flour
- ½ teaspoon garlic powder, divided
- ½ teaspoon paprika, divided
- Salt and freshly ground black pepper, to taste
- 2 large eggs, beaten
- 1 tablespoon unsweetened almond milk
- ½ cup unsweetened flaked coconut
- ¼ cup pork rinds, crushed
- ½ pound large shrimp, peeled and deveined
- Nonstick cooking spray

Directions::

1. Place the flour, half the spices, salt, and black pepper in a shallow dish and blend well.
2. Place the eggs and almond milk in a second shallow dish and beat well.
3. Place the coconut, pork rinds, remaining spices, salt, and black pepper and blend well.
4. Coat shrimp with flour mixture, then read egg mixture and eventually coat with the coconut mixture.
5. 5 Again, dip in the egg mixture and coat with the coconut mixture.

6. 6 Turn the "Temperature Knob" of PowerXL Air Fryer Grill to line the temperature to 380 degrees F.
7. 7 Turn the "Function Knob" to settle on "Air Fry."
8. 8 Turn the "Timer Knob" to line the Time for 8 minutes.
9. 9 After preheating, arrange the shrimp into the greased air fry basket.
10. Insert the air fry basket at position 2 of the Air Fryer Grill.
11. Flip the shrimp once halfway through.
12. When the cooking Time is over, transfer the shrimp onto a platter.
13. Serve immediately.

Nutrition: Calories: 234 Kcal, Fat: 13.8g, Carb, 5.9g, Protein: 20g